GET HEALTHY
STAY HEALTHY
& LIVE
for Men

Janet A. Cooksey

All scripture quotes are from the King James Version (KJV) unless otherwise noted.

Design Director: Janet A. Cooksey

ISBN-10: 1726043851
ISBN-13: 978-1726043854

WHAT'S INVOLVED
COMMITMENT, DESIRE, FAITH, BELIEF, BRAVERY, FORTITUDE & GRACE

- cardio training
- weekly weight ins
- time management
- better nutrition
- weight training
- support from group

HOW WE DO IT
GODLY DETERMINATION

- Weekly Empowerment call in
- Challenge Schedule & Program
- Prayer & Fasting
- Prayer Declarations and Daily Journaling
- Communion Daily
- Testimonies

EATING YOUR WAY TO A HEALTHY LIFESTYLE BY KICKING THE DEVIL OUT!

TABLE OF CONTENTS

90 Day Challenge to Get Healthy, Stay Healthy & Live for Men

INTRODUCTION

First, I would like to thank you for taking the opportunity to allow this program to help change your life. I believe that you will never be the same. This will be a lifestyle change, not a diet! And surely, not a quick fix!

This may be the most extraordinary transformation program ever done. Why, first we put God first. We will start each day by turning to our first love. By asking the Lord Jesus Christ for grace for our transformation: spirit, soul and body.

The focus will not be directly on weight loss but getting rid of emotional triggers, pain, deep hurt, anything that is causing harm and hurt to us spiritually, emotionally, mentally, socially, physically, physiologically, psychologically, relationally and financially. There maybe other areas that are healed during this process as well, therefore not limiting to the list above.

DISCLAIMER

Before starting this program please seek the advice of your physician. The participant assumes full responsibility for consulting a qualified health professional regarding health conditions or concerns.

This program is not intended to diagnose, treat, cure or prevent any disease. This should not be considered a substitute for professional medical expertise or treatment. The writer(s) and publisher(s) of this program are not responsible for adverse reactions, effects, or consequences resulting from any suggestions herein or procedures undertaken hereafter.

Please document all of this as well in your journal and keep daily records.

Any participant that wants to be highlighted on 90 Day Challenge FB page must send a before and after photo and a testimony of your journey.

QUESTIONS
Questions you should ask yourself before starting this program.
- How do you see yourself?
- Why do I need to do this?
- What are my goals to be completed during this program?
- How much weight do I need to lose?
- How many inches do I need to lose in (arms, thighs, abdomen, chest)?

90 Day Challenge to Get Healthy, Stay Healthy & Live for Men

- What has been your major hindrance to losing weight before?
- How do you handle stress in your life?
- How do you handle trauma and change in your life?
- Have I dealt with any issues of unforgiveness, regret, and bitterness?
- Have I dealt with any abuse in my life and how it triggers me to eat?
- Have I dealt with any offense that may have caused me to gain weight overnight?
- What medical conditions do I have that may limit me physically?
- What medications do I take that cause weight gain and any negative side effects?

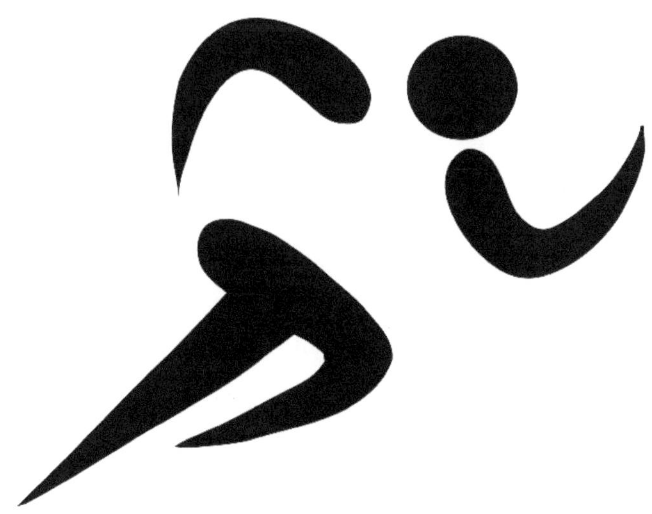

90 Day Challenge to Get Healthy, Stay Healthy & Live for Men

COMMITMENT STATEMENT

On this _________day of

__________________________________.

I ____will be truthful and honest to myself and others about how I am doing and feeling during this process.

- I choose to follow the tips and guidelines in "Eating Your Way to a Healthy Lifestyle by Kicking the Devil Out."

- I choose to be determined to achieve my goals.

- I choose to face my deepest fears.

- I choose to let go of the past to move into the present and future.

- I choose to forgive.

- I choose life, love, peace and joy.

- I choose to transform my mind, body, soul and spirit.

- I choose to stay focused.

90 Day Challenge to Get Healthy, Stay Healthy & Live for Men

- I choose to live.

- I choose to release all negativity from my soul.

- I choose to think good, pure, lovely thoughts above myself and who I am.

90 Day Challenge to Get Healthy, Stay Healthy & Live for Men

PROGRAM STRUCTURE

- *Prayer Declarations* is from Chapter 2 in Eating Your Way to a Healthy Lifestyle by Kicking the Devil Out!

- *Progressive Fast* will to get rid of the cravings for carbs and sugars and help the body to detoxify and get rid of the toxins in the body and organs, specifically the liver and cleansing the digestive system. This fast you will progressive eliminate something from your consumption and cannot consume eating it until the entire fast is over. After the fast make sure the gradually add meals back into consumption. My suggestion is to do the fast in reverse if need be. Not adding all things that you were delivered from of course.

- Resetting the *frequencies* in your body.

- *Communion* will help you to commune with the Lord each day and have a deeper relationship with the Lord Jesus Christ. Know what the finished work of cross has done for you and appropriate that in your life. (You can use eggs, bread, juice, etc.) It's the symbol, what it represents not the elements you use. I sometimes use my meals as a symbol as well.

90 Day Challenge to Get Healthy, Stay Healthy & Live for Men

- *Opening* your heart and gateways for the King of Glory to come in: Cleansing your spirit, soul and body. To explain this I use the plumbing pipe as an example. The pipe can become clogged with all types of debris that sticks to the pipe in layer upon layer where the pipes have not been cleanse in years, until there is a backup or overflow of what is in it comes up to the surface. That's what happens in our lives; we don't know what is in there until something triggers an overflow of what has been clogging us. We will uncover in each week areas that maybe clogging our heart and gateways so you can be free of those things.

1st week – Getting rid of anything that deals with anger.
2nd week – Getting rid of fear, any form of fear
3rd week – Getting rid of feelings of abandonment & rejection
4th week – Getting rid of shame
5th week – Getting rid of lying
6th week – Getting rid of financial lack, poverty
7th week – Getting rid of addictions and addictive behavior
8th week – Getting rid of sensuality

90 Day Challenge to Get Healthy, Stay Healthy & Live for Men

9th week – Getting rid of depression
10th week – Getting rid of grief
11th week – Getting rid of mental instability
12th week – Getting rid of pride
13th week – Getting rid of procrastination

- **Weekly Empowerment and Call-in** – Every Saturday morning at 8:00 AM EST or Sunday Evening 7:00 PM EST via Uberconference. You will receive confirmation and link for sessions via email. During these sessions there will be a time of prayer and impartation. Sharing testimonies and weekly status. Encouragement for each participant. Calls will be recorded and each participant will have access to the replay later. This is only for members who have paid program fee.

- **Get a tape measure to measure**: arms, chest, waist, abdomen and thighs

- **Before and After Photos** – Take (3) recent photos and (3) after photos at home: frontal, side profile, and back profile. This is for your personal journal and testimony.

90 Day Challenge to Get Healthy, Stay Healthy & Live for Men

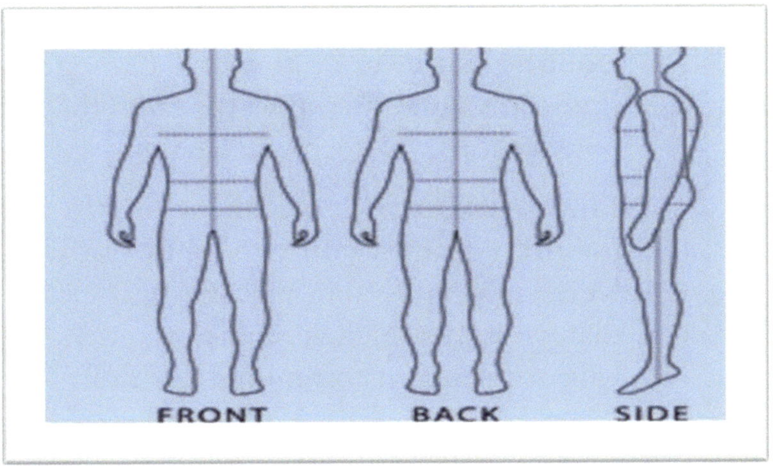

- **Writing Down Your Goals Weekly** – Take the time each week to capture or journal your goals. What do you want to achieve during each week and why do want to achieve your goal(s). Use the goal sheet at the end of program packet or use your journal. Remember if you don't complete your goal during each week, continue to press to complete it don't give up. Even if you complete 50% in that week that is awesome, keep going until it is totally completed. I'm here to say to you 5%, 10% is better than 0%. What is more important is that you give all your effort, give the best that you have and don't ever quit.

- **Determine if this is for weight loss or for transformation.**

90 Day Challenge to Get Healthy, Stay Healthy & Live for Men

- **Make sure to keep this fun and exciting experience for you.** During this find some comedy shows to watch that are positive that will keep you laughing.

- **Find workout videos that will help and inspire you that you can work out with.** Keep it simple and realistic and believe that you can achieve the goals that you have written and committed to fulfill.

There maybe modifications and updates where applicable during the transformation program.

To get the most out of this program it best advised that you use the *"Eating Your Way to a Healthy Lifestyle by Kicking the Devil Out!"* series (Book & Journal) which are available for purchase Amazon and Createspace and also directly from Author Janet Cooksey, contact at authorjanetcooksey@gmail.com.

Let's Get Started! Let's Get Moving!

Frame up your reality each day, by speaking this over your life: *Acts 17:28 For in Him we live, and move, and have our being: as certain also of your own poets have said, For we are also his offspring.* "In the name of Jesus, I speak to my body and soul (mind, will and emotions) to come under my spirit today. My spirit is under the Holy Spirit and I submit all to Jehovah God. I present my body, brain, heart, soul, spirit, imagination, all of my gateways, thoughts, attitudes, habits, behaviors, reason centre, my past, present, future as living sacrifice holy and acceptable to you Lord which is my reasonable service to You"

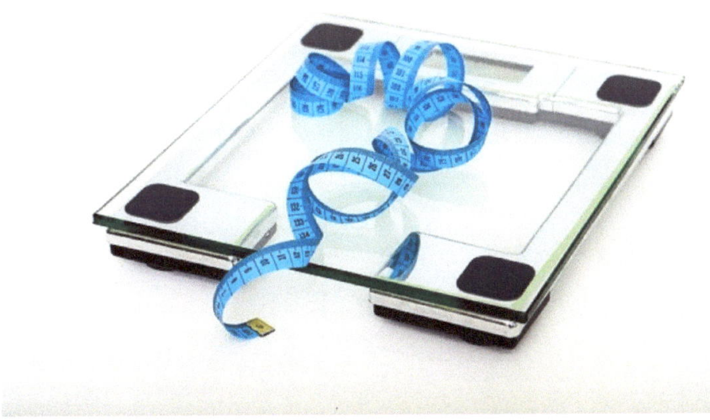

90 Day Challenge to Get Healthy, Stay Healthy & Live for Men

CALCULATING YOUR BODY MASS INDEX (BMI)

Weight/Measure	BMI
Healthy Weight	19 – 24.9
Overweight	25 – 29.9
Obese	30 and above

The Body Mass Index (BMI) is used to determine whether you are at a healthy weight or overweight. This correlates to the total fat on your body. So, calculate your BMI at every weigh-in.

How to calculate your BMI:

One of the resources you can use online to calculate your BMI is: http://www.smartbmicalculator.com/ This calculator computes the body mass index and rates it appropriately for men, women, children, juveniles and seniors, now also for Asian users.

If you prefer doing it manually here are the steps.

1. Convert your weight from pounds to kilograms
Let's say your weight is 275 Lbs and height is 6' 3"

Your weight (in pounds) ÷ 2.2 = your weight (in kilograms). For example, 275 pounds ÷ 2.2 kilograms = 125 kilograms.

2. Convert height from inches to meters.
Your height (in inches) ÷ 39.37 = your height (in meters). For example, 75 inches ÷ 39.37 meters = 1.9 meters.

3. Calculate your Body Mass Index.
Your weight (in kilograms) ÷ [your height (in meters) x your height (in meters)] = BMI. For example, 125 kilograms ÷ (1.9 meters /1.9 meters) = 34.62.

HOW TO GET YOUR BODY MEASUREMENTS

Use your cloth tape measure to take your measurements. Take your measurements on your bare skin not over clothes.

Chest: Measure the circumference of your chest. Place one end of the tape measure at the fullest part of your bust; wrap it around (under your armpits, around your shoulder blades, and back to the front) to get the measurement.

Waist: Measure the circumference of your waist. Use the tape to circle your waist at your natural waistline, which is located above your belly button and below your rib cage. Don't suck in your stomach, or you'll get a false measurement.

Hips: Measure the circumference of your hips. Start at one hip and wrap the tape measure around your rear, around the other hip, and back to where you started. Make sure the tape is over the largest part of your buttocks.

Upper arm: Measure the circumference of your arm. Wrap the tape measure around the widest part of your upper arm from front to back and around to the start point.

Body	Measurements	Body	Measurements
Before 90 Day Challenge	**After 90 Day Challenge**		
Upper Arm		*Upper Arm*	
Chest		*Chest*	
Waist		*Waist*	
Hips		*Hips*	
Thigh		*Thigh*	
Weight		*Weight*	
BMI		*BMI*	
Dress Size		*Dress Size*	

90 Day Challenge to Get Healthy, Stay Healthy & Live for Men

PROGRAM 90 DAY SCHEDULE

<table>
<tr><td>Week One</td></tr>
</table>

Focus: *first week* is *getting rid of any area of anger.*

Anger includes the following: anger, hatred, malice, rage, murder, temper, cursing, vengeance, resentment, regret, retaliation, violence, abuse, cruelty, sadism, unforgiveness, bitterness, being judgmental, taking offense easily, irritable, anger towards men, anger towards women, anger towards mother or father, anger towards authority, anger towards God, resentment towards God, anger towards yourself, unforgiveness towards yourself.

Fast Day 1: Refrain from drinking fruit drinks, sodas, energy drinks and coffee. Refrain from eating for at 3 hours.

Exercises:

Basic: *Home Workout – 15 minute walking workout for weight loss* **and great tips.**

Fast Day 2: Refrain from drinking fruit drinks, sodas, energy drinks and coffee. Refrain from eating for at 3 hours. **REST DAY**

Fast Day 3: Refrain from drinking fruit drinks, sodas, energy drinks and coffee. Refrain from eating for at 3 hours. **REST DAY**

Fast Day 4: Refrain from eating any fried foods and fast foods. Refrain from eating for at 3 hours.

Exercise:

Treadmill: 1 mile

Fast Day 5: Refrain from eating any fried foods and fast foods. Refrain from eating for at 3 hours.

Exercise:

90 Day Challenge to Get Healthy, Stay Healthy & Live for Men

Fast Day 6: Refrain from eating any fried foods and fast foods. Refrain from eating for at 3 hours.

Exercise:

Fast Day 7: Refrain from eating any sweets, candy, cakes and any type of chips. Fast by giving up 1 of your normal meals.

Exercise:

Take Communion every day

Cleanse your gateway – first love gateway, revelation, reverence

Do your Daily Declarations to Speak Over Your Body, can also do these while walking or exercising.

Before starting Weight yourself in the morning. Journal it Daily journal.

Meal Plan: Plan your meals and snacks for the week.

Week Two

Focus: *second week* is *getting rid of any fear, any form of fear.*

All Fear, worry, anxiety, fear of man, doubt, unbelief, fear of authority, dread, panic attacks, fear the worst will happen, hope deferred, fear of sickness and disease, fear of rejection, fear of failure, fear of success, spirit of false responsibility, fear of demons, fear of future

Fast Day 8: Refrain from eating any sweets, candy, cakes and any type of chips. Fast by giving up 1 of your normal meals.

Exercise:

90 Day Challenge to Get Healthy, Stay Healthy & Live for Men

Fast Day 9: Refrain from eating any sweets, candy, cakes and any type of chips. Fast by giving up 1 of your normal meals. **REST DAY**

Fast Day 10: Refrain from eating any meat. Fast by giving up 1 of your normal meals. **REST DAY**

Fast Day 11: Refrain from eating any meat. Fast by giving up 1 of your normal meals.
Exercise:
Bike: 2.5 miles

Fast Day 12: Refrain from eating any meat. Fast by giving up 1 of your normal meals.
Exercise:
Treadmill: 1.5 miles

Fast Day 13: Refrain from eating any type of dairy products. Fast by giving up 1 of your normal meals.
Exercise:
Stretching

Fast Day 14: Refrain from eating any type of dairy products. Fast by giving up 1 of your normal meals.
Exercise:
Bike: 2.5 miles

Take Communion every day

Cleanse your gateway – first love gateway, fear of God, hope

Do your Daily Declarations to Speak Over Your Body, can also do these while walking or exercising.

Before starting Weight yourself in the morning. Journal it Daily journal.

Meal Plan: Plan your meals and snacks for the week.

Week Three

Focus: *third week* is *getting rid of any area of*

90 Day Challenge to Get Healthy, Stay Healthy & Live for Men

abandonment & rejection:

Abandonment, desertion, divorce, rejection, neglect, victimization, blocked intimacy, not valuing others, not valuing relationships, not ending relationships, burning bridges, isolation, loneliness, self-pity

Fast Day 15: Refrain from eating any type of dairy products. Fast by giving up 1 of your normal meals. **Exercise:**
Treadmill: 1.5 miles

Fast Day 16: Eat only soups and light salads, light breads, fruit, and pasta. Fast by giving up 2 of your normal meals.
REST DAY

Fast Day 17: Eat only soups and light salads, light breads, fruit, and pasta. Fast by giving up 2 of your normal meals.
REST DAY

Fast Day 18: Eat only soups and light salads, light breads, fruit, and pasta. Fast by giving up 2 of your normal meals. **Exercise:**
Walk Away the Pounds – 1 Mile

Fast Day 19: Eat only soups. You may drink water and juice. Fast by giving up 2 of your normal meals. **Exercise:**
Line Dance for 15 minutes

Fast Day 20: Eat only soups. You may drink water and juice. Fast by giving up 2 of your normal meals. **Exercise**
Stretching

Fast Day 21: Eat only clear soup, water and juice only. **Exercise:**
Cardio Training

Take Communion every day

90 Day Challenge to Get Healthy, Stay Healthy & Live for Men

Cleanse your gateway – first love gateway, faith, worship

Do your Daily Declarations to Speak Over Your Body, can also do these while walking or exercising.

Before starting Weight yourself in the morning. Journal it Daily journal.

Meal Plan: Plan your meals and snacks for the week.

Focus: *fourth week* is *getting rid of any area of shame & guilt.*

Shame, anger, condemnation, disgrace, embarrassment, guilt, hatred, self-hate, self-pity, withdrawal, hiding, antisocial, timidity, inferiority

Fast Day 22: Eat only clear soup, water and juice only.
Exercise:
Weight Training

Fast Day 23: Eat only clear soup, water and juice only.
REST DAY

Fast Day 24: Drink water only. Refrain from eating any food. REST DAY

Fast Day 25: Drink water only. Refrain from eating any food.
Exercise:
Abs Workout

Fast Day 26: Drink water only. Refrain from eating any food.
Exercise
Low Intensity Cardio

Fast Day 27: Drink water only. Refrain from eating any food.
Exercise:

90 Day Challenge to Get Healthy, Stay Healthy & Live for Men

Fast Day 28: Drink only clear soup, water and juice only. **Exercise:**
Walk Away the Pounds – 2 miles
Take Communion every day
Cleanse your gateway – first love gateway, prayer, intuition
Do your Daily Declarations to Speak Over Your Body, can also do these while walking or exercising.
Before starting Weight yourself in the morning. Journal it Daily journal.
Meal Plan: Plan your meals and snacks for the week.
Week Five
Focus: *fifth week* is *getting rid of any area of lying:* Lying, cheating, theft, deception, trickery, untrustworthiness, adultery, emotional adultery, denial, self-deception, secretiveness, hiding purchases, hiding activities, hiding relationships
Fast Day 29 Drink only clear soup, water and juice only. **Exercise:** Line Dance
Fast Day 30: Drink only clear soup, water and juice only. REST DAY
Day 31: REST DAY
Day 32: **Exercise:** Shadow Boxing
Day 33: **Exercise:** Treadmill: 2 Miles

Day 34:
Exercise:
Stretching

Day 35:
Exercise:
Walk Away the Pounds – 3 Miles

Take Communion every day

Cleanse your gateway – first love gateway, imagination, conscience

Do your Daily Declarations to Speak Over Your Body, can also do these while walking or exercising.

Before starting Weight yourself in the morning. Journal it Daily journal.

Meal Plan: Plan your meals and snacks for the week.

Week Six

Focus: *sixth week* is *getting rid of any area of financial lack, poverty.*

Financial lack, poverty (belief in poverty), mammon, robbing God by not tithing, not believing in covenant blessings, greed, covetousness, debt, dishonesty, idolatry of possessions, idolatry of money, failure, parax

Note: My suggestion in regards to resuming eating is to do the fast in reverse if need be. So that your body do not go into shock, specifically your digestive system and liver.

Day 36
Exercise:
Bike: 3 Miles

Day 37: REST DAY

Day 38: REST DAY

Day 39:

Exercise:
Treadmill: 2.5 Miles

Day 40:
Exercise:
Walking Away the Miles – 3 Miles

Day 41:
Exercise:
Stretching

Day 42
Exercise:
Shadow Boxing

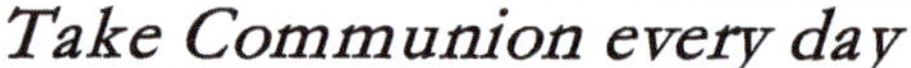

Take Communion every day

Cleanse your gateway – first love gateway, reason, mind (heart)

Do your Daily Declarations to Speak Over Your Body, can also do these while walking or exercising.

Before starting Weight yourself in the morning. Journal it Daily journal.

Meal Plan: Plan your meals and snacks for the week.

Week Seven

Focus: *seventh week* is *getting rid of any area of addictions and addictive behavior.*

Addictions, alcohol, tobacco, drugs, food, sugar, coffee, chocolate, sweets, pornography, sex, flirtation, junky magazines, social media, internet, websites, TV shows, magazines, movies, overeating, drinking too much alcohol, overindulgence in anything

Day 43:
Exercise:
Weight Training

90 Day Challenge to Get Healthy, Stay Healthy & Live for Men

Day 44: REST DAY

Day 45: REST DAY

Day 46:
Exercise:
Jump Rope

Day 47:
Exercise:
Weight Training

Day 48:
Exercise:
Stretching

Day 49:
Exercise:
Weight Training

Take Communion every day

Cleanse your gateway – first love gateway, conscious, subconscious

Do your Daily Declarations to Speak Over Your Body, can also do these while walking or exercising.

Before starting Weight yourself in the morning. Journal it Daily journal.

Meal Plan: Plan your meals and snacks for the week.

Week Eight

Focus: *eighth week* is *getting rid of any area of sensuality.*

Sensuality, lust, fantasizing, coveting another's mate, flirtation, premarital sex, sexual abuse, fornication, adultery, emotional adultery, demonic sex, pornography, bondage, control, rape, incest

Day 50:

90 Day Challenge to Get Healthy, Stay Healthy & Live for Men

Exercise: Jump Rope
Day 51: REST DAY
Day 52: REST DAY
Day 53:   *Exercise:*   Weight Training
Day 54:   *Exercise:*   Jump Rope
Day 55:   *Exercise:*   Stretching
Day 56:   *Exercise:*   Jump Rope
Take Communion every day
Cleanse your gateway – first love gateway, unconscious, emotions
Do your Daily Declarations to Speak Over Your Body, can also do these while walking or exercising.
Before starting Weight yourself in the morning. Journal it Daily journal.
Meal Plan: Plan your meals and snacks for the week.
Week Nine
Focus: *ninth week* is *getting rid of any area of depression*:
Depression, rejection, despair, helplessness, hopelessness, sadness, self-pity, withdrawal, suicide.
Day 57:

90 Day Challenge to Get Healthy, Stay Healthy & Live for Men

Exercise:
Weight Training

Day 58: REST DAY

Day 59: REST DAY

Day 60:
Exercise:
Line Dance

Day 61:
Exercise:
Treadmill – 3 miles

Day 62:
Exercise:
Stretching

Day 63:
Exercise:
Bike – 3.5 miles

Take Communion every day

Cleanse your gateway – first love gateway, will, choice

Do your Daily Declarations to Speak Over Your Body, can also do these while walking or exercising.

Before starting Weight yourself in the morning. Journal it Daily journal.

Meal Plan: Plan your meals and snacks for the week.

Week Ten

Grief, sorrow, despair, discouragement, disappointment, heartbreak, loss, pain, deep hurt, torment, weeping, anguish, agony

Day 64:
Exercise:
Line Dance

90 Day Challenge to Get Healthy, Stay Healthy & Live for Men

Day 65: REST DAY
Day 66: REST DAY
Day 67: *Exercise:* Bike- 4 miles
Day 68: *Exercise:* WATP – 4 miles
Day 69: *Exercise:* Stretching
Day 70: *Exercise:* WATP- 3 miles
Take Communion every day
Cleanse your gateway – first love gateway, eye (sight), nose (smell)
Do your Daily Declarations to Speak Over Your Body, can also do these while walking or exercising.
Before starting Weight yourself in the morning. Journal it Daily journal.
Meal Plan: Plan your meals and snacks for the week.
Week Eleven
Focus: *eleventh week* is *getting rid of any area of mental instability.*
Mental instability, mental illness, compulsions, confusion, hysteria, paranoia, schizophrenia, insanity
Day 71: *Exercise:* Bike – 5 miles

90 Day Challenge to Get Healthy, Stay Healthy & Live for Men

Day 72: REST DAY

Day 73: REST DAY

Day 74:
Exercise:
Shadow Boxing

Day 75:
Exercise:
Abs Workout

Day 76:
Exercise:
Stretching

Day 77:
Exercise:
Abs Workout

Take Communion every day

Cleanse your gateway – first love gateway, mouth (taste)

Do your Daily Declarations to Speak Over Your Body, can also do these while walking or exercising.

Before starting Weight yourself in the morning. Journal it Daily journal.

Meal Plan: Plan your meals and snacks for the week.

Week Twelve

Focus: *twelfth week* is *getting rid of any area of pride*:

Pride, arrogance, disdain, selfishness, control, manipulation, pushiness, must have your way, independence, callousness, lack of concern for others

Day 78:
Exercise:
Shadow Boxing

Day 79: REST DAY

Day 80: REST DAY

Day 81:
Exercise:
Treadmill – 4 miles

Day 82:
Exercise:
Weight Training

Day 83:
Exercise:
Stretching

Day 84:
Exercise:
Weight Training

Take Communion every day

Cleanse your gateway – first love gateway, hands (touch)

Do your Daily Declarations to Speak Over Your Body, can also do these while walking or exercising.

Before starting Weight yourself in the morning. Journal it Daily journal.

Meal Plan: Plan your meals and snacks for the week.

Week Thirteen

Focus: ***thirteenth week*** is *getting rid of any area of procrastination*:

Procrastination, slothfulness, laziness, distraction, confusion, lack of focus, lack of vision, not thinking things through before acting, speaking or writing posts, blogs, or e-mails, lack of organization, lack of preparation, lateness, tardiness, (no time management), missing appointments, missing phone calls or not responding to important phone calls

Day 85:
Exercise:
Treadmill – 4 miles
Day 86: REST DAY
Day 87: REST DAY
Day 88:
Exercise:
Weight Training
Day 89:
Exercise:
Shadow Boxing
Day 90:
Exercise:
Stretching
Take Communion every day
Cleanse your gateway – first love gateway, ear (hearing)
Do your Daily Declarations to Speak Over Your Body, can also do these while walking or exercising.
Before starting Weight yourself in the morning. Journal it Daily journal.
Meal Plan: Plan your meals and snacks for the week.

COMMUNION PRAYER

- Original Prayer by Mike Parsons, Freedom Apostolic Ministries, LTD - Modified by Janet Cooksey

- I thank you Heavenly Father for sending your only begotten son, Jesus Christ of Nazareth to redeem mankind.

- I thank you for the three-fold redemption of my spirit, soul and body, through Christ's sufferings.

- I bless this bread and wine that represent the body of Jesus Christ and the precious blood of Jesus.

- As I eat these elements I appropriate the finished work of the cross.

- As I take this I am transformed and I am becoming one with You Jesus Christ.

- I engage and partake in the DNA of God as I eat your flesh and drink your blood so that I will not die but live forever.

- I thank You that every record of sin, iniquity and transgression is dealt with. That every root of anger, fear, confusion, rebellion and every seed of the enemy: Cain seed, Nephilim seed, reptilian seed, alien seed, occultic seed, and every negative seed.

- I embrace and receive the transforming power of the body and blood of Jesus

90 Day Challenge to Get Healthy, Stay Healthy & Live for Men

- I engage the record containing the light, sound and frequency of God's image for transfiguration
- I embrace the record of the dimensions of the kingdom released in my body by the DNA of God
- I engage that DNA record and apply it to my bones for health and wholeness to remove all negative epigenetic hereditary switches
- I speak to my marrow and command it to be a new source of blood that will transform the DNA of my cells so that I can be transfigured and live forever
- I apply the frequency of God's DNA to transform me into the image of Jesus
- I command every genetic record to be transformed and my DNA to be resequenced into alignment with my eternal image
- I apply the blood of Jesus to transform all impure genetic material - be transformed
- I apply the blood of Jesus to all iniquitous genetic patterns - be cleansed
- I call all my genetic material to resonate with the DNA of God and come into alignment with my eternal image
- I choose to bear the record, my eternal image conformed to the likeness of my Father and Brother in heaven, and to be transfigured to radiate their glory

90 Day Challenge to Get Healthy, Stay Healthy & Live for Men

- Let the breath of God be breathed into my life, transforming me into a living being, joined to the Lord and one spirit with Him
- I speak creative words to my DNA to release the supernatural abilities of God
- I trigger the ability to see and move in the spiritual realm of the kingdom
- I trigger the ability to transform matter and control light and sound
- I thank you that every record of the enemy is burned up by the fire of God. As I partake Your light, your creative light is manifested in and through me
- As I receive communion Yeshua, fill me with Your love, Your life, Your fire and most of all Your being, in Yeshua's Holy name. Amen.
- Now take eat and drink!

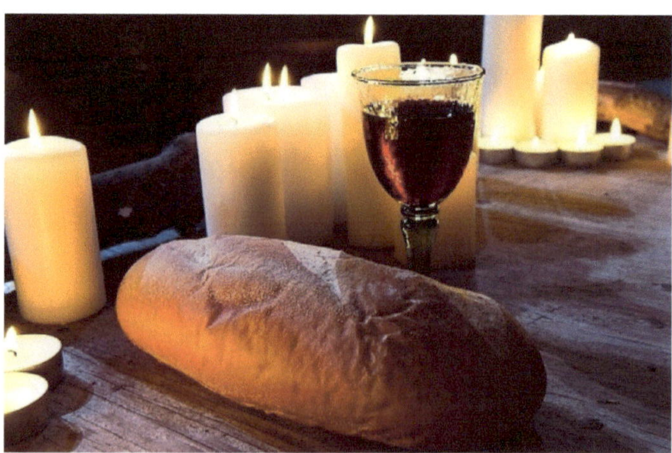

HOW TO DEAL WITH ACIDOSIS AND WHAT ARE THE SYMPTOMS

Acidosis - is an increased acidity in the blood and other body tissue. Acidosis is said to occur when arterial pH falls below 7.35. The pH level of our blood affects every cell in our body. Chronic acidosis corrodes body tissue, and if left unchecked, will interrupt all cellular activities and functions.

Sleeplessness	Headaches
Confusion	Vomiting
Diarrhea	Nausea
Coughing	Increased Heart Rate
Shortness of Breath	Arrhythmia
Loss of Consciousness	Coma
Sensation of dizziness	General feeling of weakness
Tongue is coated with a thin white layer	

KEEP YOUR BOWELS CLEANSED

Use Epsom salt solution to trigger bowel movement	May use daily enema to help eliminate toxins from the body
Colonic –bowel irrigation can also be done prior to program or during	Magnesium Citrate or Mag7 can also be used for bowel discharge.

90 Day Challenge to Get Healthy, Stay Healthy & Live for Men

WORKOUT SCHEDULE

Table Legend

WT – Weight Training	W – Walking
LD – Line Dance	LIC – Low Intensity Cardio
AW – ABS Workout	CT - Cardio Training
SB – Shadow Boxing	JR – Jump Rope
TM - Treadmill	B - Bike
S - Stretching	WI – Weigh In
RD – Rest Day	CI – Call In
WO – Weight Out	R – Running
J - Jogging	

90 Day Challenge to Get Healthy, Stay Healthy & Live for Men

Month 1						
Sunday	**Monday**	**Tuesday**	**Wednesday**	**Thursday**	**Friday**	**Saturday**
					1 WI 15 minute workout	2 RD CI
3 RD	4 TM – 1 mile	5 B – 2 miles	6 S	7 TM-1 mile	8 WI Bike – 2 miles	9 RD CI
10 RD	11 B – 2.5 miles	12 TM – 1.5 miles	13 S	14 B – 2.5 miles	15 WI TM – 1.5 miles	16 RD CI
17 RD	18 W – 1 mile	19 LD – 15-30 min.	20 S	21 CT	22 WI WT	23 RD CI
24 RD	25 AW	26 LIC	27 S	28 W-2 miles	29 WI LD – 15-30 min.	30 RD CI
31 RD						

90 Day Challenge to Get Healthy, Stay Healthy & Live for Men

Month 2						
Sunday	Monday	Tuesday	Wednesday	Thursday	Friday	Saturday
	1 SB	2 TM– 2 miles	3 S	4 W-3 miles	5 WI Bike – 3 miles	6 RD CI
7 RD	8 TM – 2.5 miles	9 W-3 miles	10 S	11 SB	12 WI WT	13 RD CI
14 RD	15 JR	16 WT	17 S	18 WT	19 WI JR	20 RD CI
21 RD	22 WT	23 JR	24 S	25 JR	26 WI WT	27 RD CI
28 RD	29 LD	30 TM– 3 miles	31 S			

90 Day Challenge to Get Healthy, Stay Healthy & Live for Men

Month 3						
Sunday	Monday	Tuesday	Wednesday	Thursday	Friday	Saturday
				1 B – 3.5 miles	2 WI LD	3 RD CI
4 RD	5 B – 4 miles	6 WATP-4 miles	7 S	8 W-3 miles	9 WI B – 5 miles	10 RD CI
11 RD	12 SB	13 AW	14 S	15 AW	16 WI SB	17 RD CI
18 RD	19 TM– 4 miles	20 WT	21 S	22 WT	23 WI TM – 4 miles	24 RD CI
25 RD	26 WT	27 SB	28 S	1	2	3 WO CI

90 Day Challenge to Get Healthy, Stay Healthy & Live for Men

WEEKLY GOAL SHEET

Week	Weekly Goals	Comp	% Comp
Week 1	Goal 1. _________________________	Yes/No	
	Goal 2. _________________________	Yes/No	
	Goal 3. _________________________	Yes/No	
	Goal 4. _________________________	Yes/No	
	Goal 5. _________________________	Yes/No	
Week 2	Goal 1. _________________________	Yes/No	
	Goal 2. _________________________	Yes/No	
	Goal 3. _________________________	Yes/No	
	Goal 4. _________________________	Yes/No	
	Goal 5. _________________________	Yes/No	
Week 3	Goal 1. _________________________	Yes/No	
	Goal 2. _________________________	Yes/No	
	Goal 3. _________________________	Yes/No	
	Goal 4. _________________________	Yes/No	
	Goal 5. _________________________	Yes/No	
Week 4	Goal 1. _________________________	Yes/No	
	Goal 2. _________________________	Yes/No	
	Goal 3. _________________________	Yes/No	
	Goal 4. _________________________	Yes/No	
	Goal 5. _________________________	Yes/No	
Week 5	Goal 1. _________________________	Yes/No	
	Goal 2. _________________________	Yes/No	
	Goal 3. _________________________	Yes/No	
	Goal 4. _________________________	Yes/No	
	Goal 5. _________________________	Yes/No	
Week 6	Goal 1. _________________________	Yes/No	
	Goal 2. _________________________	Yes/No	
	Goal 3. _________________________	Yes/No	
	Goal 4. _________________________	Yes/No	
	Goal 5. _________________________	Yes/No	
Week 7	Goal 1. _________________________	Yes/No	
	Goal 2. _________________________	Yes/No	
	Goal 3. _________________________	Yes/No	
	Goal 4. _________________________	Yes/No	
	Goal 5. _________________________	Yes/No	

90 Day Challenge to Get Healthy, Stay Healthy & Live for Men

Week 8	Goal 1. _________________________	Yes/No	
	Goal 2. _________________________	Yes/No	
	Goal 3. _________________________	Yes/No	
	Goal 4. _________________________	Yes/No	
	Goal 5. _________________________	Yes/No	
Week 9	Goal 1. _________________________	Yes/No	
	Goal 2. _________________________	Yes/No	
	Goal 3. _________________________	Yes/No	
	Goal 4. _________________________	Yes/No	
	Goal 5. _________________________	Yes/No	
Week 10	Goal 1. _________________________	Yes/No	
	Goal 2._________________________	Yes/No	
	Goal 3. _________________________	Yes/No	
	Goal 4._________________________	Yes/No	
	Goal 5. _________________________	Yes/No	
Week 11	Goal 1. _________________________	Yes/No	
	Goal 2. _________________________	Yes/No	
	Goal 3. _________________________	Yes/No	
	Goal 4. _________________________	Yes/No	
	Goal 5. _________________________	Yes/No	
Week 12	Goal 1._________________________	Yes/No	
	Goal 2. _________________________	Yes/No	
	Goal 3. _________________________	Yes/No	
	Goal 4._________________________	Yes/No	
	Goal 5. _________________________	Yes/No	
Week 13	Goal 1. _________________________	Yes/No	
	Goal 2.	Yes/No	
	Goal 3. _________________________	Yes/No	
	Goal 4. _________________________	Yes/No	
	Goal 5. _________________________	Yes/No	

ABOUT THE AUTHOR

Janet A. Cooksey is an author, speaker, life coach and executive who loves to build up "Champions!" No matter what sphere of influence you find yourself in, whether ministry or business, she has the balanced wisdom to put you on track to fulfilling your life goals. She loves to see everyone healed, whole and walking in freedom, fulfilling God-given dreams along the way.

Janet is available for speaking engagements upon request. She can be reached at RaphaHeartMinistries@gmail.com for information regarding resources, itinerary, or to schedule a ministry appointment.

For business appointments contact Janet at SavvyIntelSolutions@gmail.com for life coaching for career and business development support and resources.

On the personal side, Janet has one wonderful son and resides in the Baltimore-Washington Metropolitan Region.

Also from Janet Cooksey

Eating Your Way to a Healthy Lifestyle: by Kicking the Devil Out!

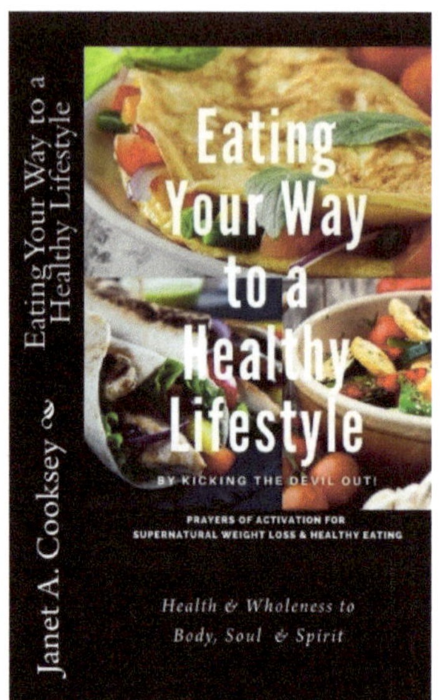

ISBN-13: 978-1973835721 (CreateSpace-Assigned)
ISBN-10: 197383572X
BISAC: Health & Fitness / Weight Loss
This book serves as a jumpstart to supernatural weight loss and a lifestyle of healthy eating.

Areas that is covered in this book is:
- Maintaining the pH -potential for hydrogen balance of the body
- Why have an alkaline diet
- Tips to increase the alkaline in your body
- What foods to eat
- How to check your pH balance
- Sample meal plan to get you started
- Daily Journal to track your progress daily
- Recipes to start with or add to your meal plans
- Prayer of Activation Supernatural Weight loss
- Daily Declarations to encourage you everyday and speak over yourself for 7 days.

30 Day Journal of Eating Your Way to a Healthy Lifestyle: by Kicking the Devil Out!

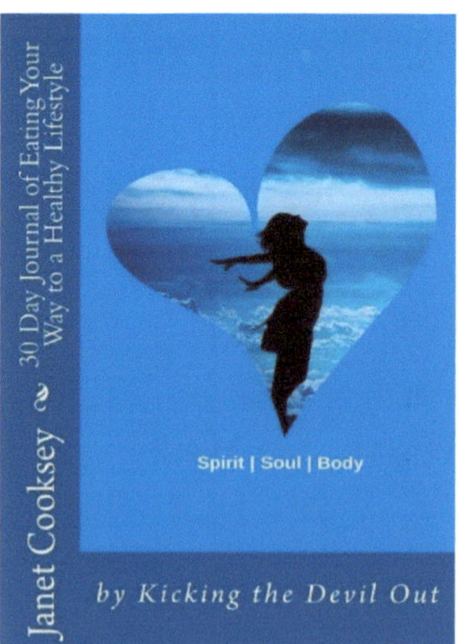

ISBN-13: 978-1979424455 (CreateSpace-Assigned)
ISBN-10: 1979424454
BISAC: Health & Fitness / Healthy Living

This journal will help you to capture your daily food choices, habits and exercise patterns. It will help you to make habitual changes to help with supernatural weight loss and eating healthy. It will help you identify triggers that contribute to reaching for carbohydrates, sugary foods and eating without being hungry. Helps to identify what you are eating when you are under pressure, stressed and anxious. It is in the series of Eating Your Way to a Healthy Lifestyle and by Kicking the Devil Out!

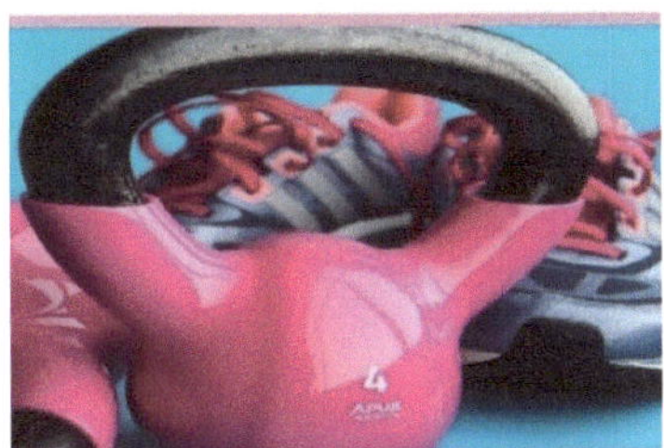

90 Day Challenge: Get Healthy Stay Healthy & Live
ISBN-13: 978-1981220410
ISBN-10:1981220410

This may be the most extraordinary transformation program ever done. Why, first we put God first. We will start each day by turning to our first love. By asking the Lord Jesus Christ for grace for our transformation: spirit, soul and body.

The focus will not be directly on weight loss but getting rid of emotional triggers, pain, deep hurt, anything that is causing harm and hurt to us spiritually, emotionally, mentally, socially, physically, physiologically, psychologically, relationally and financially. There maybe other areas that are healed during this process as well, therefore not limiting to the list above.

30 Day Journal to a Healthy Lifestyle for Men
ISBN-10: 1726045978
ISBN-13: 978-1726045971

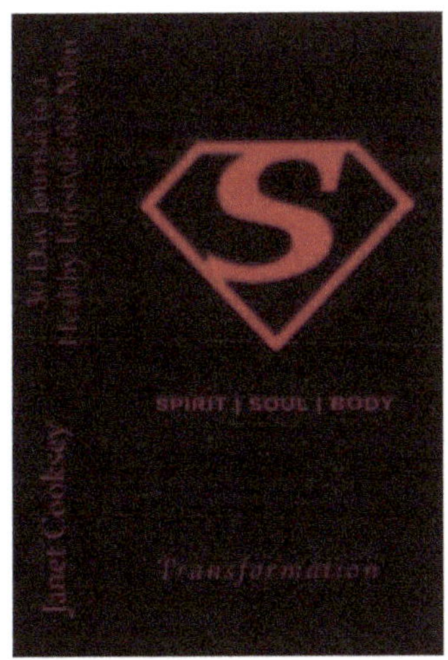

This journal will help you to capture your daily food choices, habits and exercise patterns. It will help you to make habitual changes to help with supernatural weight loss and eating healthy. It will help you identify triggers that contribute to reaching for carbohydrates, sugary foods and eating without being hungry. Helps to identify what you are eating when you are under pressure, stressed and anxious. It is in the series of Eating Your Way to a Healthy Lifestyle and by Kicking the Devil Out!. You will be able to record: -Daily Journal of your food and beverages, breakfast, lunch, dinner, and snacks. -Capture your weight each day. -Capture your exercises. -Journal how your emotions throughout the day to help identify triggers. -Includes Daily Declarations and biblical scriptures for daily meditation with an impartation of the anointing for supernatural weight loss and the breaker anointing upon your life within this series.